# EMPOWERED MENOPAUSE FOR WOMEN

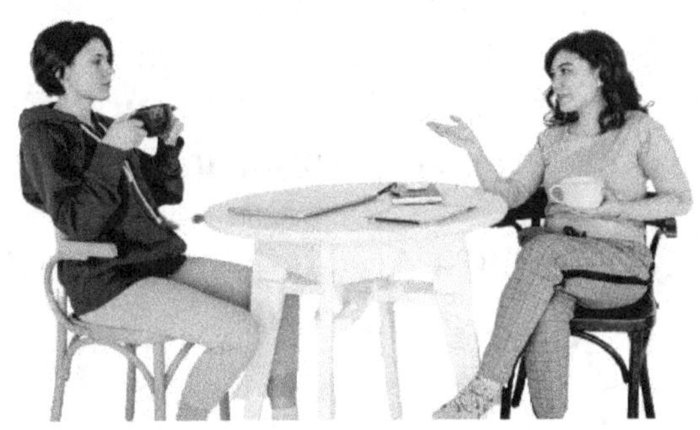

## *A TO Z GUIDE FOR THRIVING THROUGH THE TRANSITION*

## ANGELA K. BUTLER

# DISCLAIMER:

The information contained in this book is for informational purposes only and is not intended to be a substitute for professional advice. While every effort has been made to ensure the accuracy of the information presented, Angela K. Butler and the publisher assume no responsibility for errors or omissions, or for the results obtained from the use of this information. Readers are encouraged to seek professional guidance for their specific needs.

# TABLE OF CONTENTS

# CHAPTER 1:
# INTRODUCTION

## 1.1: Understanding Menopause

Throughout most of my life, my period was always there. Sometimes it came with cramps and bloating, other times it was just a quiet part of life. It was like a clock ticking in the background, always reliable. But as I got older, around my late forties, things started to change. My period wasn't as regular anymore. Sometimes it would skip months, then surprise me by showing up unexpectedly. It felt strange, like a friend suddenly acting differently.

One busy morning, as I scrambled to find a tampon and reorganize my day, I felt frustrated. "Is this how things are going to be?" I wondered, imagining a future filled with hot flashes and less energy. The idea of menopause, which had always seemed far away, suddenly felt very real. But then, I remembered something from when I was younger.

When I was a teenager, I loved ballet and read everything I could about the famous dancers. I read about Margot Fonteyn, who kept dancing even in her fifties. She broke the stereotype of older dancers slowing down. She kept getting better with age.

Remembering this made me realize something important. Menopause isn't the end of the story; it's just a new beginning. Yes, my body is changing, but that doesn't mean my life is over. And that's what I want to tell you – menopause isn't a decline; it's a chance to start something new. It's a natural change that lets us redefine what it means to be a woman as we move into this exciting stage of life.

## 1.2: Understanding Hormonal Changes in Menopause

Remember those awkward days of your first period in middle school? Suddenly, your body started acting unpredictably – mood swings, sudden growth spurts, and maybe even a hot flash (hopefully not in front of your crush!). Well, menopause can feel a bit like that – a hormonal shift that disrupts your once-familiar system. But unlike adolescence, menopause is a natural transition, and knowing the science behind it can empower you to navigate it smoothly (and perhaps with less sweating!).

Think of our bodies like complex orchestras, with the brain as the conductor, sending signals to different sections (organs and glands) to keep everything in harmony. During our reproductive years, our ovaries are the main players in this hormonal symphony. These small powerhouses in our lower abdomen produce hormones like estrogen and progesterone. Estrogen acts as the lead violinist, regulating our menstrual cycle, bone health, and mood. Progesterone, like the oboe, supports estrogen, thickening the uterine lining for pregnancy.

Now, imagine this: for years, your ovaries have conducted this hormonal symphony flawlessly. Then, around your late 40s or early 50s, things start to change. The egg supply dwindles, like musicians retiring from an orchestra. Estrogen and progesterone production declines – the lead violinist's melody falters, and the oboe's notes weaken. This hormonal imbalance leads to menopausal symptoms.

Let me share Sarah's story. A fitness enthusiast and life of the party, Sarah noticed changes around 48. Night sweats disrupted her sleep, her energy dipped, and mood swings became the norm. It was like her reliable body had become a stranger.

Thankfully, Sarah took action. Learning about hormonal changes in menopause was eye-opening. "It all clicked!" she said. Understanding why her sleep suffered and her emotions fluctuated helped her regain control.

She adjusted her diet, added estrogen-boosting foods like flaxseed, and started calming yoga for stress relief and better sleep. Gradually, she felt like herself again.

Understanding menopausal biology, like Sarah did, is key to taking charge of your health. The decline in estrogen and progesterone may change the tune, but you can actively participate. By making adjustments, you can create your own vibrant and empowered menopausal experience.

## 1.3: Understanding The Stages And What to Expect During Each Stage

Let's be real, ladies, the word "menopause" can sound a bit old-fashioned, like a cheese puff left out too long. But here's the deal: menopause isn't the end; it's a change. Think of it as a new beginning, a chance to redefine what it means to be a strong, vibrant woman.

Before you think it's all downhill from here, hold up! Menopause isn't just one big event. It's like a play with different parts: perimenopause, menopause, and postmenopause.

## Part 1: Perimenopause - The Warm-Up

Imagine driving along life's road, your periods always on time, when suddenly, things get unpredictable.
Your cycle goes haywire – sometimes longer, sometimes shorter. That's perimenopause. It's like a warm-up to the main event, usually starting in your 40s and lasting a few years.

For me, perimenopause was sneaky. One moment, I was myself, the next, I was hunting for tampons because of a surprise period. And those hot flashes? Picture being in an important meeting and suddenly feeling like you're in an oven. Explaining that to colleagues was quite the challenge.

But here's the good part: perimenopause gets you ready. It's your body's way of getting ready for big changes. Even though the symptoms can be annoying, they're a sign that things are changing.

## Part 2: Menopause - The Big Change

Ah, menopause. It's when your periods stop for a whole year. This is like Act 2 of the play.

This phase can last different amounts of time. Some women have symptoms from perimenopause that stick around, while others feel better pretty quickly. It depends on your own story.

## Part 3: Postmenopause - Enjoying the Ride

Once you've gone a year without a period, congratulations! You're in postmenopause. This is the longest part, lasting the rest of your life.

But you know what? It's often the best part. Many women feel free in postmenopause. No more worrying about periods or mood swings. You're in charge, free to live life your way.

**The Takeaway**
Remember, these stages are like a map, not rules. Your experience will be unique. Some women have an easy time, while others find it harder. But knowing what to expect is the first step to making menopause a positive change.

So, when you think of "menopause," don't see it as an end. Picture a strong woman ready for a new chapter, filled with wisdom, strength, and endless possibilities.

# CHAPTER 2: YOUR MENOPAUSE, YOUR EXPERIENCE

Think back to that slightly old cheese puff I mentioned earlier. That's how I felt when I first noticed the changes. It was as if someone had flipped a switch inside me, and suddenly everything felt... different. My periods, once predictable, became unpredictable guests, showing up whenever they wanted (or not at all). And those hot flashes – oh, the hot flashes! One moment I'd be fine, and the next I'd be sweating as if I had just completed a marathon in the Sahara.

It was all so bewildering! They call it menopause, but what does that really mean for **me**? That's when I realized the most important lesson about this entire journey: **my menopause, my story.**

## 2.1 Identifying Your Symptoms and Timeline

Menopause, a word often whispered with some uncertainty, marks a significant shift in a woman's life. It signifies the end of her reproductive years, but more importantly, it introduces a new phase filled with opportunities.

However, the journey to menopause varies for each woman. Every woman experiences this transition differently, with her own set of symptoms and timeline. Understanding these differences is crucial for embracing your personal journey through menopause.

## A Range of Symptoms

While the cessation of menstruation is the most recognized symptom of menopause, it often comes with various physical and emotional changes. Some women may encounter mild disruptions, while others may face more pronounced symptoms. Here's an overview of the potential experiences:

1. **Physical Symptoms:** Changes in menstrual patterns, hot flashes and night sweats, vaginal dryness, alterations in sleep patterns, weight fluctuations, decreased libido, urinary urgency or incontinence, hair thinning or loss, dry skin and eyes.
2. **Emotional Symptoms:** Mood swings, irritability, anxiety, depression, difficulty focusing, memory issues.

It's important to note that not all women will experience every symptom, and the severity can vary greatly.

Some may find their symptoms manageable, while others may require medical support to find relief.

## Recognizing Symptoms

The first step in navigating your menopause journey is to **recognize the symptoms**. Pay attention to your body's signals. Are your menstrual cycles becoming irregular? Have you noticed sudden heat waves followed by chills? Do you wake up sweating excessively at night? These could indicate the onset of perimenopause, the phase leading up to menopause.

Keeping a **symptom journal** can be helpful. Record the date, type of symptom, and its intensity. This can assist in locating trends and possible triggers. For instance, you might notice that hot flashes occur more often during times of stress or after consuming certain foods.

## The Unique Timing of Menopause

Menopause doesn't happen abruptly like flipping a switch; it unfolds gradually. This transitional period, called **perimenopause**, typically lasts four to eight years, though it may vary in duration for each woman. During this time, estrogen and progesterone production gradually decreases, impacting menstrual regulation.

Menopause is officially diagnosed after a full year without menstruation. However, the journey doesn't end there. **Postmenopause** refers to the years following menstruation cessation and can last indefinitely. While some women may experience lingering symptoms, others may find hormonal stability and relief.

## Understanding Individual Differences

The timing and intensity of your menopause experience will be unique to you. Several factors, including age, genetics, lifestyle, and medical conditions, can influence your journey.

## Embrace Your Path

Menopause isn't a one-size-fits-all experience. Embrace your uniqueness. Acknowledge your distinct symptoms and timeline. Avoid comparing your journey to others', and seek medical advice if you face disruptive or concerning symptoms.

With knowledge and self-awareness, you can navigate menopause confidently. Remember, it's a natural transition, not a disease. By understanding the range of experiences and influencing factors, you can turn this phase into a positive and empowering chapter in your life.

## 2.2: Mastering Your Body's Signals

Hey, ladies, our bodies are pretty amazing at talking to us. They send signals all the time – like hunger pangs, a racing heart before a big moment, or that relaxed feeling after a good massage. But during menopause, these signals can get a bit confusing. Suddenly, we're dealing with unexpected hot flashes, mood swings that feel like a rollercoaster, and sleep patterns that seem all over the place. So, what's our body trying to say?

Well, here's the good news: with a bit of practice, we can become experts at understanding our body's unique "menopause language." Here's how:

**The Power of Mindfulness**

Imagine you're on a quiet mountaintop, feeling the breeze and focusing on your breath. That's mindfulness – being in the moment without judgment, just noticing what's happening inside you.

Mindfulness helps us understand our body's signals during menopause. By taking a few quiet moments each day to focus on our breath and how our body feels, we can start to pick up on subtle cues. Do you feel tense before a hot flash? Does certain food make you tired? The more you pay attention, the more your body will reveal.

You can practice mindfulness in different ways:
- **Meditation:** Select a peaceful area, shut your eyes, and concentrate on your breathing.
- **Deep Breathing:** Take slow, deep breaths, feeling your belly rise and fall.

- **Body Scan:** Lie down comfortably and focus on each part of your body.

## Keeping a Symptom Journal – Your Personal Menopause Guide

Think of a symptom journal like those secret decoder rings from childhood – it helps translate what your body is saying during menopause.

Here's how to create one:

- ❖ Get organized: Use a notebook or an app on your phone.
- ❖ Record details: Write down the date, time, and any symptoms. Be specific!
- ❖ Look for patterns: After a few weeks, see if any symptoms happen together or at certain times.
- ❖ Identify triggers: Your journal can help spot what makes symptoms worse.

## Embracing Your Intuition And Your Body's Whisperer

We all have that inner voice guiding us. During menopause, it's essential to listen to it.

Here's how:

1. **Trust your gut:** If something feels off, pay attention.
2. **Notice patterns:** Craving a specific food? It could be just what your body requires.

### Becoming a Body Language Pro Takes Time

Don't worry if you don't master it straight away. It takes practice and patience. But with mindfulness, a symptom journal, and listening to your intuition, you'll understand your body's messages better.

Remember, during menopause, your body is changing a lot. By learning its language, you can navigate this time with more ease and empower yourself for a healthy, fulfilling life ahead.

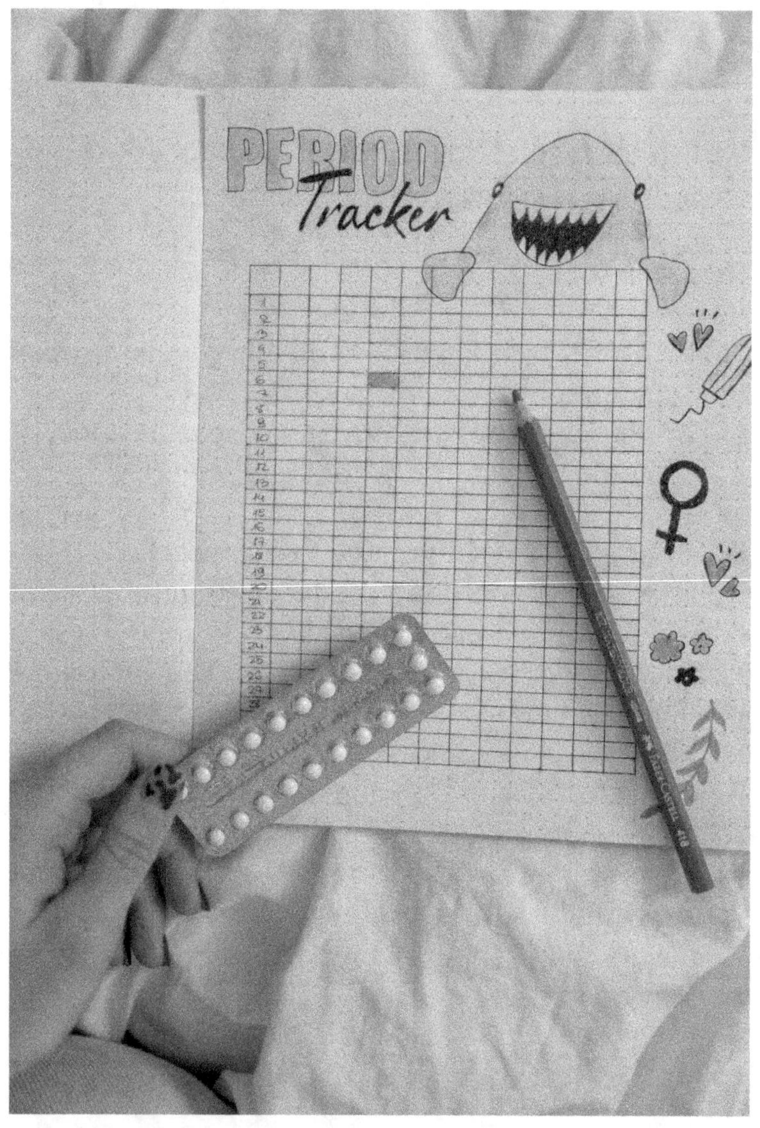


PERIOD
Tracker

# CHAPTER 3: UNDERSTANDING YOUR MENOPAUSE SYMPTOMS

Menopause is a word that often brings to mind hot flashes, mood swings, and feeling like things are spiraling out of control. While these symptoms can be tough, knowing why they happen can help women handle this phase of life better.

**How Your Hormones Work Together**
Think of your body like a big orchestra, with hormones like estrogen and progesterone as the main instruments. These hormones control lots of things, including your menstrual cycle. But during perimenopause, the time leading up to menopause, their levels start to change, going down over time.

**Estrogen: The Multitasking Hormone**

Estrogen does many jobs in your body, from keeping your bones strong to helping you feel good. But when estrogen levels drop during menopause, these jobs don't work as well, causing common symptoms like:

- Hot Flashes and Night Sweats: Less estrogen messes with your body's temperature control, leading to sudden heat and sweating.

- Vaginal Dryness: Estrogen keeps your lady parts healthy and moist, so less of it can make things dry and uncomfortable.
- Sleep Changes: Estrogen also affects your sleep, so lower levels can lead to trouble sleeping and feeling tired during the day.
- Mood Swings and Forgetfulness: Estrogen helps your brain work right, so when it changes, you might feel moody or forgetful.

## Progesterone: Estrogen's Helper

Progesterone works with estrogen to get your body ready for a possible baby. During perimenopause, progesterone levels go down too, though not as much as estrogen. This drop can make periods irregular and mood swings worse.

## Other Changes in Your Body

The drop in estrogen and progesterone doesn't just affect menopause symptoms. It can also mess with other things, like your mood and bone strength.

## Understanding Helps You Take Control

Knowing why menopause symptoms happen can help you deal with them better. For example, if you know hot flashes come from changes in estrogen, you can try things like wearing light clothes or managing stress to feel better.

And if you understand that mood swings might be because of hormones, you can be kinder to yourself and try relaxation techniques or talk to a doctor if you need help.

Understanding the science behind menopause might seem hard, but it can help you feel more confident and take better care of yourself during this time.

## 3.1: Cracking the Code of Physical Changes During Menopause

Menopause marks the end of a woman's reproductive years and often brings along a range of physical transformations. While some women sail through this phase smoothly, others find themselves facing a rollercoaster of physical ups and downs. Understanding the common physical symptoms of menopause can give women the confidence to navigate this journey more effectively.

**The Hormonal Shake-Up**

The main drivers behind the physical changes during menopause are the decreasing levels of estrogen and progesterone. These hormones are crucial for regulating the menstrual cycle and overall health.

As their levels drop, the body reacts, resulting in various physical symptoms associated with menopause.

## The Iconic Hot Flash

One of the most recognizable menopausal symptoms is the hot flash. These sudden bursts of heat can feel like a wave washing over the body, often causing sweating, flushed skin, and a racing heart. Hot flashes can disrupt sleep and daily activities but usually become less intense and frequent over time.

## Night Sweats: Hot Flashes' Nighttime Version

Night sweats are closely related to hot flashes but occur during sleep, leaving you waking up soaked in sweat. They can disturb sleep quality, leading to fatigue and irritability during the day. Like hot flashes, they're believed to result from hormonal changes affecting the body's temperature regulation.

## Other Physical Changes

Besides hot flashes and night sweats, menopause can bring about other physical shifts:

I. Vaginal Dryness: Declining estrogen levels can cause thinning and dryness of vaginal tissues, leading to discomfort and increased vulnerability to infections during intercourse.

II. Sleep Pattern Changes: Many women experience sleep problems like insomnia or waking frequently during the night, often due to hormonal fluctuations or stress.

III. Weight Changes: Some women may notice weight gain, especially around the abdomen, during menopause. Regular exercise combined with a good diet can help control weight.

IV. Bladder Issues: Hormonal changes and muscle tone fluctuations can result in urinary urgency or incontinence.

## Understanding Your Journey

Each woman's experience of menopause is unique, with symptoms varying in intensity and duration. It's essential to recognize and accept this individuality.

## Seeking Help

If you're struggling with bothersome physical symptoms during menopause, don't hesitate to consult your doctor. They can offer personalized advice, recommend effective management strategies, or discuss treatment options to help you navigate this phase more comfortably.

By understanding and addressing the physical changes that come with menopause, you can better manage your health and well-being during this transition and beyond. Recall that on this road, knowledge is your ally.

## 3.2 Navigating Mood Swings, Anxiety, and Depression During Menopause

Menopause isn't just about hot flashes and night sweats; it can also bring about emotional changes. Mood swings, anxiety, and feelings of depression can become part of your life during this time. It's essential to understand that these emotional shifts are common and not a sign of weakness. Hormonal changes, especially in estrogen and progesterone levels, are the main reasons behind these emotional ups and downs.

**Understanding Hormonal Impact**

Estrogen and progesterone play big roles in keeping our moods stable. As menopause approaches, the production of these hormones starts to decrease. This change can mess with the balance of emotions in your brain, leading to various emotional changes:

- Mood Swings: You might go from feeling happy to suddenly feeling irritable or tearful, and it can be hard to predict.
- Anxiety: Feeling more worried or nervous than usual becomes common. You might struggle to relax or enjoy things you used to.
- Depression: Experiencing feelings of sadness, hopelessness, or disinterest in things you once loved are signs of depression. It's essential to seek help if you think you're experiencing this.

## Other Influences on Emotions

Apart from hormonal shifts, other factors can affect your emotional well-being:

- Stress: Managing life's stressors can be tough during menopause when you're juggling various responsibilities.
- Lifestyle Choices: Your diet, exercise routine, and sleep patterns all impact your mood.
- Social Support: Having people to talk to and lean on can make a big difference during this time.

## Dealing with Emotional Changes

Here are some strategies to help you handle emotional changes during menopause:

I.   Educate Yourself: Knowing how hormones affect your emotions can help you recognize and manage your feelings better.

II.   Self-Care: Taking care of yourself physically and emotionally is crucial. Make sure you exercise, eat healthfully, get adequate sleep, and engage in pleasurable activities.

III.   Stress Management: Find healthy ways to manage stress, like deep breathing or spending time with loved ones.

IV.   Connect with Others: Don't keep your feelings bottled up. Speak with loved ones, friends, or a therapist.

V.   Seek Professional Help: If your emotions are overwhelming, seek help from a doctor or therapist.

Emotional changes during menopause are common, and you're not alone. By understanding what's happening, recognizing the symptoms, and using healthy coping strategies, you can navigate this phase with greater ease and continue to live a balanced life.

# CHAPTER 4: CRAFTING YOUR TREATMENT PLANS

Think of your journey through menopause like a challenging hike. You'll face ups and downs, but you're not going alone. You've got a toolbox full of strategies to help you navigate and reach your goal: a healthy, happy life.

**Exploring Treatment Options**

There's no one solution for managing menopause symptoms. Your choices depend on how severe your symptoms are, your health, and what works best for you. Here's a look at some options:

1. **Hormone Replacement Therapy (HRT):** This common treatment involves replacing the hormones your body isn't making anymore. It can help with hot flashes, night sweats, and more. But it's essential to talk to your doctor about the risks and benefits.

"I used to have intense hot flashes all the time. HRT changed everything. They became less frequent, and I felt more comfortable."

2. **Alternative Therapies:** Many women find relief through other methods like:

I. Herbal Remedies: Some herbs like black cohosh might help with symptoms, but always talk to your doctor first.

II. Acupuncture: This traditional Chinese practice can ease hot flashes and night sweats for some women.

III. Mind-Body Techniques: Practices like yoga and meditation can reduce stress and improve sleep.

"I didn't want hormones, so I tried yoga. It helped me manage stress and sleep better."

3. **Lifestyle Changes**: Simple adjustments can make a big difference:

I. Diet: Eating well supports hormone balance and overall health.

II. Exercise: Regular activity boosts mood, energy, and sleep quality.

III. Sleep Habits: Good sleep routines, like a consistent bedtime, can improve sleep.

"I changed my diet, started walking, and focused on sleep. It wasn't instant, but I felt better over time."

## Crafting Your Plan

There's no one-size-fits-all approach. Here's how to make a plan that fits you:

- Talk to Your Doctor: They can help tailor a plan to your needs and guide you through the process.
- Be Patient: Finding the right mix of treatments may take time.
- Speak Up: Don't hesitate to share your concerns and questions with your doctor.

## Your Treatment Toolbox: Your Guide to Empowerment

Your toolbox is full of options. By exploring what works for you, you can manage menopause confidently and enjoy life to the fullest.

# 4.2: A Comprehensive Look at Hormone Replacement Therapy (HRT)

Hormone Replacement Therapy (HRT) is a common term in menopause discussions, yet it often remains surrounded by uncertainty for many women. Questions arise about its effectiveness against menopausal symptoms and the associated risks. It's crucial to grasp both the benefits and risks of HRT to make an informed decision about its suitability for you.

## Understanding HRT: Replacing What's Needed

Menopause entails a decline in estrogen and progesterone production, vital hormones for menstrual cycle regulation and overall bodily functions. HRT steps in to replenish these hormones, potentially easing various menopausal symptoms.

HRT can be administered in several ways:

> ➤ Oral tablets: These are daily pills containing estrogen, progesterone, or a combination of both, the most prevalent form of HRT.
> ➤ Skin patches: Applied to the skin, these patches release hormones gradually into the bloodstream.

> ➢ Vaginal creams or gels: These localized therapies deliver estrogen directly to vaginal tissues, primarily addressing vaginal dryness and discomfort.

## A Range of Benefits

HRT offers numerous benefits for managing menopause symptoms, including:

A. **Relief from hot flashes and night sweats:** Considered the most effective treatment, HRT significantly reduces the frequency and intensity of these symptoms.
B. **Improvement in vaginal dryness and discomfort:** HRT aids in restoring moisture and elasticity to vaginal tissues, enhancing sexual function and reducing discomfort during intercourse.
C. **Alleviation of mood swings and depression:** Studies suggest HRT can ease symptoms of anxiety and depression linked with menopause.
D. **Enhancement of sleep quality:** By reducing night sweats and stabilizing mood, HRT can improve sleep patterns.
E. **Support for bone health:** Estrogen is crucial for bone health, and HRT can help prevent bone loss and lower the risk of osteoporosis in certain women.

## Key Considerations: Evaluating Risks

While HRT offers compelling benefits, understanding the potential risks is essential. These risks vary depending on the type of HRT, medical history, and individual factors. Here's a breakdown of some potential concerns:

- Breast cancer: Certain types of HRT, particularly those combining estrogen and progestin, may slightly increase the risk of breast cancer. The risk in absolute terms is still minimal, though.
- Blood clots: Some forms of HRT pose a small increased risk of blood clots, particularly for women with a history of blood clots or those at higher risk.
- Stroke: Limited research suggests a potential increased risk of stroke with certain forms of HRT.

## Making an Informed Choice

The decision regarding HRT is personal, with no definitive right or wrong answer. Here are essential steps to consider:

- → Consult Your Doctor: Seek guidance from a healthcare professional specializing in women's health to discuss your individual needs, risk factors, and the potential benefits and risks of HRT.

→ Assess Your Symptoms: The severity and types of symptoms you experience will influence the decision. If hot flashes are predominant, HRT may be a viable option.

→ Weigh Risks and Benefits: Discuss any underlying health conditions that might affect the risks associated with HRT.

→ Explore Alternatives: If HRT isn't suitable for you, explore alternative treatment options, such as lifestyle adjustments or complementary therapies.

## HRT: Tailored to Your Needs

HRT remains a valuable tool for managing menopause symptoms, but it's not a one-size-fits-all solution. The key lies in open communication with your doctor, understanding your individual needs and risks, and collaboratively devising a personalized plan for navigating menopause and maintaining overall well-being.

# 4.2: Exploring Alternatives: Herbal Remedies and Personalized Approaches

Alright, ladies, let's chat about choices. We all know Hormone Replacement Therapy (HRT) is a common option for managing menopause symptoms. But what if HRT isn't right for you? Don't fret! There's a world of alternative therapies waiting for you to explore, kind of like stepping into a lively farmers market full of natural remedies and holistic practices.

**Harnessing Nature's Wisdom: Herbal Solutions**

For centuries, women have turned to nature for support during menopause. Here are some herbal options you might consider:

- Black Cohosh: This herb is known to reduce hot flashes and night sweats, but it's essential to talk to your doctor first.
- Red Clover: With compounds similar to estrogen, red clover may help with symptoms like vaginal dryness and mood swings, but always consult your doctor before trying it.
- Evening Primrose Oil: This oil might improve skin health and ease vaginal dryness,

but again, speak with your doctor before adding it to your routine.

**Important Reminder:** While herbs offer potential benefits, they're not a quick fix. Results may vary, so consulting a qualified herbalist or naturopathic doctor is wise to ensure they're safe and suitable for you.

## Acupuncture: Balancing Your Energy Flow

A mainstay of traditional Chinese medicine, acupuncture involves the insertion of tiny needles into certain body sites. Research suggests it can help manage hot flashes and night sweats by stimulating the nervous system and regulating hormone production.

**Personal Experience with Acupuncture:** Initially skeptical, I tried acupuncture for my hot flashes. Surprisingly, it was relaxing! After a few sessions, I noticed a decrease in the intensity and frequency of my hot flashes.

## Mind-Body Harmony: Yoga, Meditation, and Mindfulness

Menopause can be stressful, but mind-body practices offer relief:

- Yoga: Combining postures, breathing exercises, and meditation, yoga enhances strength, mood, and stress reduction.
- Meditation: Spending a few minutes daily to focus on your breath can alleviate stress and anxiety.
- Mindfulness: Being present without judgment helps manage emotional ups and downs.

**Crafting Your Personal Plan: Tailored Support**

Alternative therapies can be combined for a personalized approach:

1. Consult a Professional: Partner with a healthcare provider versed in alternative therapies for guidance.
2. Start Slow: Introduce one or two therapies at a time to gauge their impact.
3. Listen to Your Body: Pay attention to how your body reacts, and adjust your plan accordingly.

There's no one-size-fits-all solution for menopause. Be patient, explore alternatives, and design a plan that empowers you to navigate this transformative phase with confidence and well-being.

# CHAPTER 5: THE ESSENTIAL PILLARS OF SELF-CARE

Throughout menopause, our bodies undergo a multitude of changes. Fluctuations in hormones can impact our mood, energy levels, sleep quality, and even our relationship with food. However, the empowering reality is that you hold the ability to shape your experience during this phase. By prioritizing three fundamental pillars of self-care – nourishing your body, engaging in physical activity, and cultivating a sleep-friendly environment – you can establish a sturdy groundwork for navigating menopause and embracing the journey ahead with vitality.

## 5.1: Nourishing Your Body: Creating a Dietary Foundation for Menopause

Let's face it, managing a healthy diet can sometimes feel like a constant battle. We struggle with cravings, resist the temptation to skip breakfast, and navigate a world full of tempting snacks. Menopause can add a new layer of challenges to this mix.

Personally, I found myself grappling with cravings for sugary treats and experiencing constant fatigue. However, I discovered that by making simple yet effective changes to my diet, I could significantly enhance my energy levels and overall well-being.

The empowering news is that you have the ability to turn your diet from a source of frustration into a cornerstone for a successful menopause journey. By embracing a dietary approach centered on whole foods, you can supply your body with the vital nutrients it requires to navigate this hormonal shift with resilience and vigor.

## Key Approaches To Constructing Your Dietary Foundation

Imagine your plate as a canvas bursting with colors. Here are the essential elements you should integrate to craft a dietary masterpiece for menopause:

- **Prioritize Whole Foods:** Fill your plate with nature's colorful bounty – fruits, vegetables, and whole grains. These nutrient-packed powerhouses supply your body with vital vitamins, minerals, and fiber. Fiber helps promote satiety, aids in digestion, and can help stabilize blood sugar levels, which may fluctuate during menopause.

**Expert Tip:** Aim for a minimum of five servings of fruits and vegetables daily, ensuring a diverse range of colors to maximize nutrient intake. For long-lasting energy, choose whole grains like oats, brown rice, quinoa, and whole-wheat bread.

- **Reduce Processed Foods:** Beware of packaged snacks and convenience meals loaded with added sugars, unhealthy fats, and excess sodium. These components may cause weight gain and exacerbate certain menopause symptoms, such as hot flashes and mood swings.

**Keep in Mind:** You're not denying yourself; you're making informed decisions to nourish your body. Instead of reaching for processed snacks when cravings strike, opt for a piece of fruit paired with almonds. Your taste buds may need time to adjust, but your body will appreciate the change.

- **Embrace Healthy Fats:** Healthy fats, found in avocados, fatty fish, nuts, and seeds, are valuable allies during menopause. They play a vital role in hormone regulation, cellular function, and promoting satiety. Including healthy fats in your diet can help regulate appetite, enhance satiety, and uplift your mood.

**Expert Tip:** Incorporate a source of healthy fats into each meal and snack. Add olive oil to vegetables, include sliced avocado on toast, or enjoy a handful of mixed nuts for a satisfying snack.

- **Stay Hydrated:** Water is essential, especially during menopause. Adequate hydration aids in flushing out toxins, regulating body temperature, and sustaining energy levels. Dehydration can mimic menopause symptoms like fatigue and headaches, so it's crucial to stay hydrated.

Aim for eight glasses of water daily, adjusting based on activity levels and climate. If plain water isn't appealing, try infusing it with cucumber, lemon, or berries. Herbal teas are also excellent hydrating options.

## Constructing Your Customized Plate And Tailoring Your Diet

These strategies form the foundation for a robust dietary plan during menopause. However, remember that everyone's body is unique. Here are additional tips for personalizing your diet:

➢ Listen to Your Body:
Pay attention to how foods impact your well-being.

Do sugary treats leave you drained? Do spicy foods trigger more hot flashes? Keeping a food journal can help identify triggers and adjust your diet accordingly.

➢ Consult a Dietitian:

A registered dietitian can craft a personalized meal plan tailored to your needs and preferences during menopause. They can also offer guidance on managing any dietary restrictions you may have.

➢ Experiment with New Foods:

Explore new recipes and discover nutritious ingredients that you enjoy. The world of delicious and wholesome foods is waiting to be explored!

## 5.2 : The Impact of Physical Activity on Menopause

Let's be real, exercising wasn't always my top priority. Sure, I understood its benefits, but the idea of sweating it out at the gym never really appealed to me. However, once menopause hit, and my energy levels plummeted while my mood swings soared, I discovered the transformative power of moving my body. Regular physical activity became a game-changer, not just for my fitness but for my overall well-being.

During menopause, our bodies undergo significant changes. Hormonal fluctuations can leave us feeling sluggish, irritable, and utterly drained. However, here's the silver lining: exercise emerges as a potent tool for managing these symptoms and fostering a happier, healthier version of ourselves.

## Elevating Mood through Movement

Ever heard of endorphins? These natural feel-good chemicals flood your brain during exercise, contributing to that post-workout high. It's not just about physical achievement; it's your brain rewarding you with a dose of happiness. This endorphin release can substantially uplift your mood and counteract the emotional turbulence often associated with menopause.

## Stress Reduction and Enhanced Sleep with Exercise as Your Ally

In today's fast-paced world, stress is a constant companion, exacerbated by the additional anxieties of menopause. However, exercise stands as a formidable stress reliever. Physical activity helps clear your mind, release tension, and foster feelings of tranquility. Consequently, this promotes restful sleep, a challenge for many women during menopause. Regular exercise facilitates faster sleep onset, deeper sleep, and enhanced morning vitality.

## Building a Resilient, Thriving You: The Multifaceted Benefits of Exercise

The advantages of exercise extend beyond mood enhancement and improved sleep quality. Consider these additional reasons to embrace physical activity during menopause:

❖ Weight Control: Menopause often triggers metabolic shifts, making weight management more challenging. Exercise aids in calorie expenditure, facilitating weight maintenance and overall well-being.

❖ Fortifying Bones: Bone density loss is a concern for menopausal women. Weight-bearing exercises like walking, running, or dancing strengthen bones, mitigating the risk of osteoporosis, especially crucial as estrogen levels decline.

❖ Boosting Confidence: Regular physical activity fosters self-esteem. As you enhance your fitness and strength, you'll likely notice a positive shift in body image and overall confidence.

## Discovering Your Exercise Style

Let's face it; spending hours on a treadmill may not ignite joy for everyone. The key to sustainable exercise lies in finding activities you genuinely relish. Here are some ideas to get you going on your journey:

A. Embrace Outdoor Activities: Take a nature walk, cycle with friends, or embark on a leisurely hike. Fresh air and sunlight can invigorate your mood.

B. Dance Freely: Put on your favorite tunes and dance your heart out! Dance classes offer a joyful way to elevate your heart rate and unleash your inner dancer.

C. Join Fitness Communities: Explore various fitness classes like yoga, Pilates, or Zumba. Group workouts provide motivation and camaraderie.

D. Home-Based Workouts: Utilize free online workout videos or design your own routine using bodyweight exercises.

**Remember:** Even short bursts of activity throughout the day yield significant benefits. Begin at your own pace, gradually increasing intensity and duration. Exercise ought to be an enjoyment of your body's abilities rather than a penalty.

So, don your favorite workout attire, engage in an activity you adore, and get moving! Your mood, sleep, and overall well-being will reap the rewards.

## 5.3: Crafting Your Sleep Haven And Establishing Serenity for Restful Nights

Let's face it, ladies, achieving a restful night's sleep can feel elusive during menopause. One moment you're drifting into slumber, the next you're battling hot flashes at 3 am. These nocturnal disruptions, coupled with stress and anxiety, can throw your sleep patterns off balance. However, fear not! By cultivating a dedicated **sleep sanctuary** and embracing calming routines, you can reclaim those precious hours of rest and wake up feeling rejuvenated and prepared to tackle the day ahead.

**Identifying Sleep Disruption Factors**

Menopause introduces several factors that can impede sleep quality. Here's what to watch out for:

- **Hormonal Changes:** Fluctuations in estrogen and progesterone, formerly the guardians of your sleep cycle, can disrupt both falling asleep and staying asleep.

- **Hot Flashes and Night Sweats:** Sudden spikes in body temperature can startle you awake and leave you feeling uncomfortable and damp.
- **Stress and Anxiety:** Life's stressors, amplified during menopause, can hinder relaxation and hinder the transition into sleep.

## Crafting Your Sleep Sanctuary

Your bedroom should serve as a tranquil refuge conducive to restorative sleep. Consider these suggestions to transform your space:

I. Temperature Management: Maintain a cool room temperature, ideally between 60-67°F (15.5-19.4°C), for optimal sleep. Utilize cooling fans or adjustable thermostats to regulate temperature fluctuations.

II. Light Control: Embrace darkness to promote restful sleep. Block out external light sources with blackout curtains or an eye mask.

III. Soothing Ambiance: Counteract disruptive noises with white noise machines or earplugs to cultivate a serene auditory environment.

IV. Comfort Optimization: Invest in a supportive mattress and pillows crafted from breathable materials like cotton or linen for enhanced comfort.

## Establishing a Relaxing Sleep Routine

Consistent bedtime rituals signal to your body that it's time to unwind and prepare for sleep. Include these routines in your evening routine:

❖ Set a Sleep Schedule: Maintain a consistent sleep-wake cycle by retiring and rising at consistent times daily, even on weekends.

❖ Pre-Bedtime Wind-Down: Engage in calming activities like reading, bathing, or gentle stretching to unwind at least an hour before bedtime, steering clear of stimulating endeavors like screen time.

❖ Dim the Lights: Diminish bedroom lighting an hour before bedtime to facilitate melatonin production, promoting drowsiness.

❖ Relaxation Practices: Incorporate relaxation techniques such as deep breathing, meditation, or light yoga to quiet the mind and induce a tranquil state conducive to sleep.

❖ Moderate Consumption: Limit intake of caffeine and alcohol, as these substances can disrupt sleep patterns, hindering restfulness.

Establishing a sleep sanctuary and nurturing calming routines demand patience and consistency. Embrace the journey and remain steadfast, acknowledging that results may require time to manifest.

## Advanced Sleep Strategies

- Regular Exercise: Incorporate moderate physical activity into your routine to enhance sleep quality, avoiding vigorous exertion close to bedtime.
- Stress Management: Combat stress with healthy coping mechanisms like yoga, meditation, or nature immersion to promote relaxation.
- Dietary Considerations: Avoid heavy meals and sugary snacks before bed, opting instead for light, nourishing options that support sleep onset.
- Medical Consultation: If sleep disturbances persist despite lifestyle adjustments, seek guidance from a healthcare professional to address potential underlying issues.

By cultivating a sleep sanctuary and integrating these practices, you can reclaim restful slumber and awaken each morning revitalized and prepared to embrace the day with renewed vigor and positivity throughout your menopause journey!

# CHAPTER 6: A COMPREHENSIVE STRATEGY FOR MANAGING SYMPTOMS AND ENHANCING INTIMATE WELLNESS

Menopause is a natural progression, yet it often accompanies a slew of unwelcome symptoms and alterations in intimate experiences. However, fret not! This section equips you with a holistic strategy – the All-in-One Symptom Management and Intimate Wellness Plan. By embracing wholesome practices and delving into solutions for sexual vitality, you can traverse menopause with assurance and sustain a gratifying lifestyle.

## 6.1: Utilizing Nutrition, Physical Activity, and Sleep for Symptom Alleviation

Recall our discussion on the significance of self-care in Chapter 5? Well, this segment elucidates how embracing a wholesome lifestyle can serve as your clandestine tool for mitigating prevalent menopause symptoms. Here's how:

## 1. **Nutrition:**

Your dietary choices directly influence your body's capacity to navigate hormonal fluctuations. Prioritize a well-rounded diet abundant in fruits, vegetables, and whole grains. These nourishing foods furnish vital vitamins, minerals, and antioxidants crucial for bolstering overall health and vitality.

## 2. **Personal Insight:**

Amidst menopause, I found myself yearning for sugary indulgences incessantly, leading to lethargy. Upon integrating more fruits and vegetables into my diet, I experienced heightened energy levels and better resilience against hot flashes and mood swings.

## 3. **Physical Activity**:

Engaging in regular exercise emerges as a potent strategy for managing menopause-related symptoms. Regular physical exertion can:

a. Diminish occurrences of hot flashes and night sweats: Research indicates that exercise aids in regulating body temperature and enhancing sleep quality, thereby mitigating the frequency and intensity of hot flashes.

b. Elevate mood and vitality: Physical activity triggers the release of endorphins, neurotransmitters renowned for counteracting anxiety and depression, prevalent during menopause.

c. Sustain a healthy weight: Menopause often entails metabolic alterations, predisposing individuals to weight gain. Exercise serves as a means to regulate weight, consequently ameliorating overall health and tempering the severity of certain menopause symptoms.

4. Sleep:

Adequate sleep is imperative, particularly during menopause. Optimal rest equips individuals with the resilience to confront physical and emotional challenges. Here are some guidelines for fostering restful sleep:

a. Establish a consistent sleep routine: Adhere to a set bedtime and waking time daily, including weekends.

b. Cultivate a tranquil bedtime ritual: Indulge in soothing activities like a warm bath, reading, or gentle stretches to unwind before retiring for the night.

c. Optimize sleep surroundings: Ensure your sleep environment is conducive to rest, characterized by cool, dim, and quiet surroundings.

**Recall:** Adhering to these healthy habits consistently is paramount!
The more diligently you prioritize these practices, the better equipped you'll be to manage symptoms and embrace a more rejuvenated state throughout menopause.

## 6.2: Techniques for Sustaining a Gratifying Sexual Experience Throughout and After Menopause

Alright, ladies, let's delve into a topic that often veers into taboo territory: sexual intimacy during menopause. While it might not be the casual brunch conversation starter, sustaining a fulfilling sexual life remains integral to overall well-being. Fortunately, menopause doesn't signify the demise of intimacy! With insight and practical approaches, you can reignite the flame and continue relishing satisfying sexual encounters amid this transition and beyond.

**Navigating Menopause's Impact on Sexuality**

Menopause precipitates hormonal adjustments that can influence sexual desire and satisfaction in several ways:

- Vaginal Dryness: Diminished estrogen levels may lead to vaginal dryness and tissue thinning, rendering intercourse uncomfortable.
- Decreased Libido: Hormonal fluctuations, notably in testosterone, can contribute to a decline in sexual drive.
- Body Image Shifts: Weight fluctuations and alterations in body image might affect self-confidence, impacting sexual enjoyment.

## Communication is Paramount

Initiating candid discussions with your partner serves as the initial stride in navigating these changes. Openly addressing concerns and preferences facilitates collaborative problem-solving, fostering a mutually fulfilling sexual experience.

## Consider these communication strategies:

- ➢ Select a Serene Moment: Opt for a relaxed, distraction-free time conducive to open dialogue.
- ➢ Utilize "I" Statements: Express feelings and concerns using "I" statements to foster understanding.

> ➤ Active Listening: Attentively listen to your partner's perspectives and apprehensions without judgment.
> ➤ Focus on Resolutions: Collaboratively explore solutions tailored to individual needs and preferences.

## Reviving the Flame: Approaches for a Rewarding Sexual Journey

Recall, a satisfying sex life need not mirror that of your younger years. Menopause presents an opportunity to embrace novel avenues for intimacy. Consider these strategies:

I. Prioritize Foreplay: Devote ample time to foreplay to facilitate natural lubrication and anticipation, incorporating techniques like massage or sensual touch.

II. Experiment with Positions: Explore positions that alleviate discomfort associated with vaginal dryness, identifying those most comfortable for you.

III. Communication Amidst Intimacy: Don't hesitate to articulate needs and preferences during intercourse, ensuring a mutually pleasurable experience.

IV. Embrace Diverse Forms of Intimacy: Recognize that physical intimacy transcends penetrative sex. Foster connection through cuddling, kissing, and other non-penetrative forms of touch.

## Addressing Vaginal Dryness

Vaginal dryness is commonplace during menopause, yet viable solutions abound:

1. Utilize Lubricants: Water-based lubricants mitigate vaginal dryness, enhancing comfort during intercourse.
2. Incorporate Moisturizers: Regular application of vaginal moisturizers bolsters lubrication and tissue health. Consult your physician to ascertain safe and effective options.

## Beyond Physical Intimacy:

Acknowledge that intimacy encompasses emotional connection as well. Nurture emotional intimacy through:

- Quality Time: Engage in shared activities that foster connection and enjoyment.
- Physical Affection: Express affection through gestures like hand-holding, cuddling, or mutual massages.
- Express Gratitude: Communicate appreciation for your partner through verbal affirmations and gestures of love.

**Recall:** You're not navigating this journey solo. If grappling with sexual concerns during menopause, consult your physician. They can address underlying medical factors and proffer guidance on strategies to reignite the spark and sustain a gratifying sexual life.

By fostering transparent communication, exploring novel avenues for connection, and addressing physical challenges, you can cultivate a fulfilling and enjoyable sexual life throughout menopause and beyond. Embrace this phase as an opportunity for intimacy rekindling and fortification of your bond with your partner.

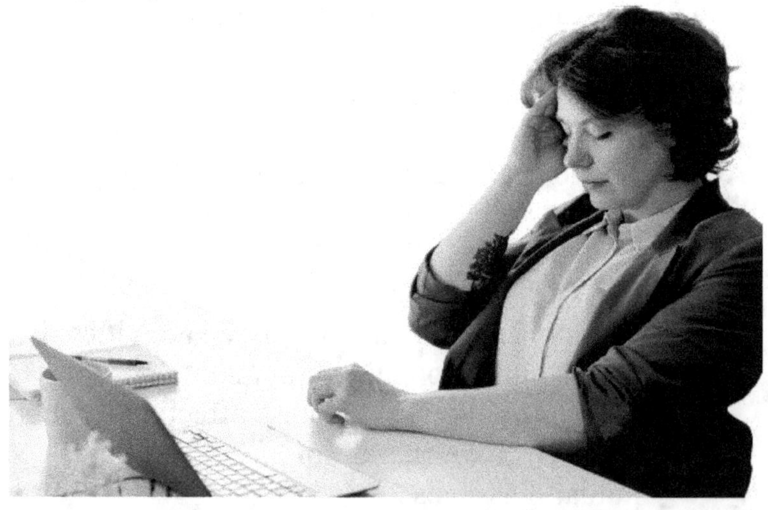

# CHAPTER 7: UNDERSTANDING AND COPING WITH EMOTIONAL CHALLENGS USING CBT

Some women liken the experience of menopause to an emotional rollercoaster. Moments of elation swiftly give way to bouts of anxiety or melancholy. These fluctuations in mood can be bewildering and daunting. However, here's the empowering reality: you're not traversing this journey alone, and there exist effective methodologies to bolster your emotional well-being amid this transition. This chapter delves into the emotional terrain of menopause and introduces Cognitive Behavioral Therapy (CBT) as a potent tool to enhance emotional resilience during this phase.

## 7.1: Addressing Mood Swings, Anxiety, and More

Menopause evokes images of physical symptoms like hot flashes, but its impact on emotions often remains unspoken. In my personal journey through menopause, I found myself riding an emotional rollercoaster.

One moment, I'd be elated, and the next, engulfed by waves of sadness or frustration. These emotional fluctuations are common during menopause, warranting an understanding of their origins and effective coping mechanisms.

**The Role of Hormones:**

The emotional landscape of menopause hinges largely on the volatile shifts in estrogen and progesterone levels. Once regulating menstrual cycles, these hormones bid adieu with erratic behavior, influencing brain chemistry and affecting mood, emotions, and cognitive function.

**Common Emotional Trials:**

Here's a closer look at some emotional challenges encountered during menopause:

A. Mood Swings: Menopause often manifests as an emotional seesaw, with abrupt bouts of irritability, tearfulness, or anger surfacing unexpectedly, disrupting daily life and relationships.

B. Anxiety: Hormonal fluctuations can induce anxiety, leading to feelings of worry, restlessness, difficulty concentrating, or physical symptoms like palpitations and breathlessness.

C. Depression: Distinguishing between occasional sadness and clinical depression is crucial. While transient low moods are typical during menopause, clinical depression entails persistent sadness, loss of interest in activities, changes in appetite or sleep, and feelings of hopelessness. Consult a doctor if these symptoms endure.

D. Brain Fog: Many women report experiencing brain fog during menopause, characterized by impaired concentration, forgetfulness, and mental sluggishness, impacting work and daily activities negatively.

Emotional challenges during menopause are neither a sign of weakness nor a personal shortcoming but a normal facet of hormonal transitions. Understanding the underlying causes can foster self-compassion and equip individuals with effective coping strategies.

## Beyond Hormones: Additional Influences on Emotional Well-being

While hormones play a pivotal role, other factors contribute to emotional distress:

- Life Stressors: Concurrent life challenges such as caring for aging parents or career transitions can exacerbate emotional fluctuations during menopause.

- Social Stigma: Enduring stigma surrounding menopause may lead to feelings of isolation and shame, exacerbating emotional struggles.

- Lack of Support: Absence of a supportive network of friends, family, or understanding healthcare professionals can amplify emotional challenges.

## Taking Charge of Emotional Well-being

Acknowledging emotional shifts during menopause and understanding contributing factors empower proactive management. Consider these strategies:

→ Open Communication: Discuss experiences with loved ones, seeking understanding and support during emotional episodes.

→ Join Support Groups: Engage with other menopausal women in support groups, fostering camaraderie and sharing coping mechanisms.

→ Seek Professional Assistance: When self-management proves challenging, seek guidance from therapists experienced in navigating menopausal emotional challenges.

You're not alone in this journey. By comprehending the emotional landscape of menopause, implementing proactive coping measures, and seeking support when necessary, individuals can navigate this phase with heightened emotional resilience, emerging stronger.

## 7.2: Leveraging Cognitive Behavioral Therapy (CBT) And Practical Strategies for Emotional Management

Amidst the challenges of menopause, there's a beacon of hope: Cognitive Behavioral Therapy (CBT), a transformative approach to managing emotional upheavals. CBT, a psychotherapeutic technique, focuses on identifying and altering negative thought patterns contributing to emotional turmoil. Let's explore how CBT can empower you:

- Challenging Negative Thought Patterns: CBT equips individuals with tools to recognize and challenge detrimental thought patterns fueling emotional distress. For instance, reframing thoughts like "I'm a failure for misplacing my keys" to "It's common to forget sometimes; I'll calmly retrace my steps" can significantly uplift mood and well-being.

- Developing Coping Mechanisms: CBT imparts practical coping mechanisms to tackle stress and anxiety, such as deep breathing, progressive muscle relaxation, and mindfulness. Mastering stress management techniques aids in navigating emotional fluctuations and maintaining serenity.

- Enhancing Communication Skills: Effective communication is pivotal, especially during menopause-induced emotional fluctuations. CBT facilitates the improvement of communication skills, fostering stronger interpersonal relationships by assertively expressing needs and feelings.

- Establishing Attainable Goals: CBT assists in setting realistic and attainable goals, fostering a sense of accomplishment and bolstering confidence. Celebrating milestones along the journey cultivates a positive outlook.

## Practical Measures For Implementing CBT in Daily Life:

Incorporate CBT principles into your daily routine with these actionable steps:

1. Identify Triggers: Recognize situations or events triggering negative emotions to develop effective coping mechanisms.

2. Challenge Negative Thoughts: When negative ideas come to mind, consider their veracity and rephrase them to seem more optimistic.

3. Practice Relaxation Techniques: Regularly engage in relaxation techniques like deep breathing and mindfulness to promote emotional calmness.

4. Set SMART Goals: Establish goals that are Specific, Measurable, Achievable, Relevant, and Time-bound to stay motivated and celebrate achievements.

5. Seek Professional Support: If managing emotions independently proves challenging, consider seeking guidance from a qualified professional.

By integrating CBT strategies into daily life, individuals can navigate the emotional landscape of menopause with resilience and empowerment.

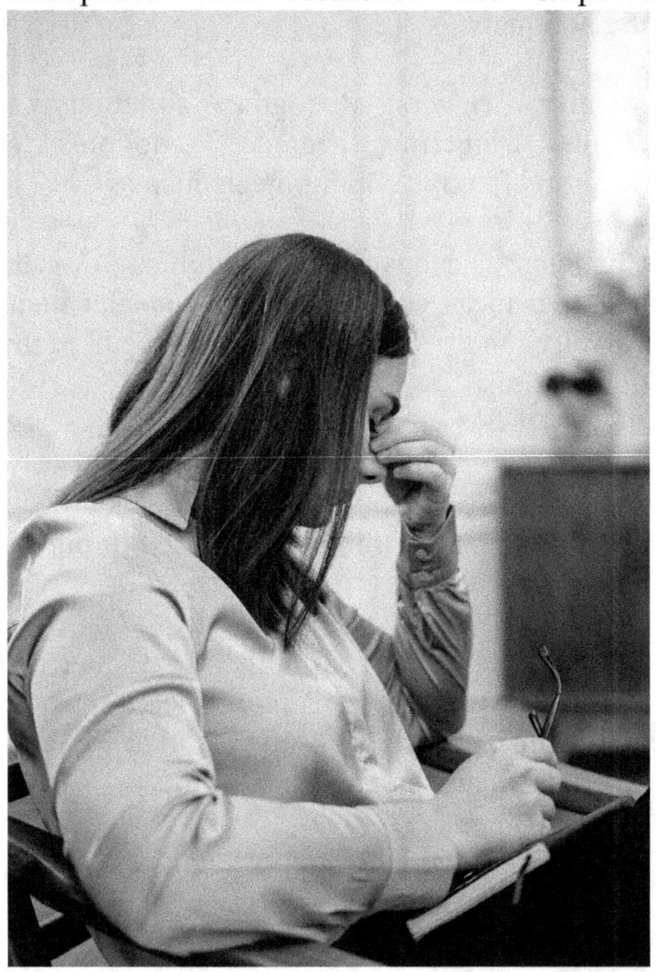

# CHAPTER 8: EVOLVING FAMILY DYNAMICS: SUSTAINING HEALTHY RELATIONSHIP

Menopause transcends mere physical changes; it intricately influences familial relationships. Reflecting on my personal journey, I observed a subtle withdrawal from social circles and a waning patience with my spouse during menopause. Interactions with my adult children seemed fraught with miscommunication, fostering concerns about our familial bond weakening. It's crucial to recognize that these challenges are widespread. However, with transparent communication, adaptive measures, and a focus on quality interactions, one can adeptly traverse these shifting family dynamics, preserving robust, nurturing relationships throughout the menopausal phase.

## Comprehending Familial Impact

Menopause casts ripples across family dynamics through various channels:

- Emotional Fluctuations: Hormonal upheavals during menopause manifest as mood swings, irritability, and fatigue, potentially straining familial communication.

- Reassessment of Priorities: Menopause prompts introspection, leading to revised priorities and altered energy levels, impacting familial engagements.
- Role Transitions: Concurrently, as children mature, familial roles naturally evolve, intertwining with menopausal adjustments, possibly engendering a sense of role ambiguity.

## Building Essential Communication

Effective communication serves as the linchpin for navigating familial transformations amid menopause. Here are strategies to foster understanding and fortify familial bonds:

- Select Apt Timing and Setting: Initiate discussions during tranquil moments, devoid of distractions, fostering receptivity and attentiveness.
- Share Personal Experiences: Candidly elucidate menopausal experiences, articulating physical and emotional challenges without dwelling on negativity.
- Emphasize "I" Statements: Express feelings and needs using "I" statements to foster empathy and circumvent accusatory tones.

- Engage in Active Listening: Encourage dialogue by attentively addressing queries and concerns sans judgment, nurturing reciprocal understanding.
- Educate Family Members: Equip loved ones with factual resources on menopause, fostering comprehension and empathy toward your experiences.

## Strengthening Familial Bonds

Having laid the foundation of open dialogue, consider strategies to fortify familial ties amid menopause:

1. Reevaluate Expectations: Collaboratively adjust expectations to accommodate shifting energy levels, fostering a sense of shared responsibility without undue burden.
2. Exemplify Empathy: Cultivate empathy by acknowledging familial concerns and perspectives, fostering cooperative problem-solving and mutual support.
3. Prioritize Quality Time: Despite diminished energy reserves, prioritize meaningful interactions, irrespective of activity, to nurture familial connection and forge cherished memories.
4. Express Gratitude: Express heartfelt appreciation for familial support and

understanding during the menopausal journey, nurturing a culture of acknowledgment and reciprocity.

By embracing transparent communication and implementing adaptive strategies, familial bonds can withstand the tumult of menopausal transitions, fostering resilience and fortitude within the family unit.

# 8.1: Discussing Menopause with Loved Ones

Broaching the topic of menopause with loved ones might initially feel uncomfortable. Throughout my own menopause journey, I hesitated to share my challenges, fearing burdening my family and unsure of their response. However, transparent communication proves indispensable in navigating the physical and emotional shifts of menopause alongside loved ones. Initiating dialogue not only fosters mutual understanding but also strengthens familial bonds, providing essential support during this phase.

**Significance of Communication**

Engaging in open discussions about menopause yields various benefits:

- Stress Alleviation: Suppressing emotions can heighten stress and anxiety; conversely, open dialogue offers emotional release and relief.
- Enhanced Relationships: Transparent communication cultivates empathy and support, enhancing relationships as loved ones gain insight into your experiences.
- Combatting Isolation: Menopause may induce feelings of isolation, yet discussing it with loved ones reinforces the sense of solidarity and offers communal support.
- Empowerment: Taking ownership of one's well-being begins with effective communication, facilitating access to vital information and support networks.

**Strategies for Communicating with Loved Ones**

Armed with an understanding of communication's importance, consider practical tips for discussing menopause with loved ones:

1. Select Appropriate Timing and Setting: Choose moments devoid of distractions, fostering conducive environments for open dialogue.
2. Share Personal Experiences: Express candidly the physical and emotional toll of

menopause, articulating challenges without dwelling on negativity.

3.  Utilize "I" Statements: Articulate feelings and needs using "I" statements to convey vulnerability and solicit support.
4.  Listen Empathetically: Be receptive to queries and concerns, offering a non-judgmental space for dialogue.
5.  Optional: Provide Education: Offer credible resources on menopause if comfortable, empowering loved ones with factual information.

Tailoring the conversation to specific individuals involves additional considerations:

- Partner Communication: Given the intimacy of the relationship, prioritize specificity regarding how symptoms affect both parties and explore collaborative solutions.
- Children Dialogue: Addressing children about menopause necessitates age-appropriate honesty, with younger children benefiting from simplified explanations and older ones engaging in deeper discussions.

Recognize that discussions may unfold gradually, with the primary objective being to initiate dialogue and sustain open communication.

## Overcoming Communication Obstacles

Anticipate and address common communication hurdles:

**Fear of Burdening:**
Embrace vulnerability and seek support, recognizing that loved ones genuinely care about your well-being.
**Embarrassment:**
Normalize menopause as a natural life phase, dispelling embarrassment and fostering acceptance.
**Knowledge Gaps:**
Offer credible resources to alleviate confusion and enhance understanding among loved ones.

# 8.2 Strengthening Family Bonds And Adapting to Changing Roles and Dynamics

Life is a perpetual cycle of change, and menopause marks a significant juncture in familial dynamics. Personally, it prompted a reassessment of my maternal role as my children transitioned into adulthood, necessitated adjustments in my relationship dynamics with my spouse, and even led to modifications in interactions with extended family members.

While these shifts may initially unsettle, they also offer an opportunity to forge deeper, more resilient connections with loved ones. Here are strategies to navigate these evolving family dynamics during menopause.

## Understanding Transformation

Menopause can influence family dynamics in several ways:

- Revised Priorities: Hormonal fluctuations may prompt shifts in priorities, leading to a desire for increased self-care or decreased energy for previous familial activities, potentially inducing feelings of guilt or disconnection.
- Evolving Roles: Transitioning from primary caregiver to a more independent parental role can evoke feelings of loss or ambiguity, while adjustments may be needed in partner relationships to accommodate physical and emotional changes.
- Communication Hurdles: Emotional fluctuations may complicate communication,

contributing to heightened impatience or withdrawal, fostering misunderstandings and tensions within the family.

## Strategies for Strengthening Bonds

By acknowledging potential shifts and approaching them proactively, one can navigate these changes and cultivate stronger familial connections.

A. Reevaluating Expectations:
Honest discussions about evolving needs and energy levels can prompt adjustments in household responsibilities, social commitments, and childcare duties, fostering a supportive familial environment. Observing my own family, my children readily assumed additional responsibilities like grocery shopping and meal preparation upon recognizing my fatigue.

B. Practicing Empathy:
Understanding and validating the emotions of family members amidst changes can foster mutual support and understanding, alleviating worries and uncertainties. Open communication and empathy are fundamental in navigating these transitions collectively.

C. Celebrating Growth:
Menopause presents an opportunity for personal growth and self-discovery. Acknowledging

individual strengths and achievements, while celebrating familial milestones, nurtures a positive and supportive environment.

D. Establishing New Traditions:

As roles evolve, creating new traditions fosters shared experiences and strengthens familial bonds. Whether through regular game nights, movie outings, or book clubs, prioritizing quality time cultivates lasting memories and connection.

E. Prioritizing Quality Time:

Despite diminished energy levels, carving out meaningful moments for family interactions is crucial. Engaging in activities tailored to current capacities, such as leisurely reading sessions or nature walks, facilitates bonding and fosters emotional closeness.

Change, though inevitable, need not be perceived negatively. By adopting a positive and proactive stance, navigating shifting family dynamics during menopause can lead to deeper connections and resilience within the familial unit.

**Bonus Tip:** Embrace Support Networks! Relying on a robust support system beyond immediate family, including friends, extended relatives, or therapists, offers invaluable emotional backing and eases the challenges of menopause transition. Cultivating a strong support network ensures access to understanding and assistance throughout this journey.

# CHAPTER 9: COMPREHENSIVE DAILY MENOPAUSE MANAGEMENT THROUGH HOLISTIC, HERBAL, AND MINDFUL PRACTICS

Menopause need not be viewed as a struggle against one's own body. Numerous women discover considerable alleviation and an enhanced feeling of wellness through the integration of holistic methodologies into their daily regimens. This chapter explores complementary treatments, herbal solutions, and mindfulness exercises, presenting a holistic approach to navigating the menopausal experience from all angles.

## 9.1: Integrative Therapies for Symptom Alleviation

Complementary therapies, also known as integrative therapies, complement traditional medicine to enhance overall wellness and target specific symptoms.

These therapies play a vital role in managing various menopause-related issues, including:

- **Hot Flashes and Night Sweats:** Among the most prevalent and disruptive menopausal symptoms, complementary therapies aid by inducing relaxation, enhancing blood circulation, and mitigating inflammation, ultimately reducing the frequency and intensity of hot flashes.
- **Anxiety and Mood Swings:** Hormonal fluctuations during menopause significantly affect mood. Complementary therapies offer a natural approach to managing anxiety, fostering emotional balance, and enhancing sleep quality, indirectly uplifting mood.
- **Sleep Disturbances:** Many women experience difficulty sleeping during menopause. Complementary therapies promoting relaxation and stress reduction significantly improve sleep quality.
- Pain Management: Some women experience joint pain and muscle aches during menopause. Certain complementary therapies provide relief by reducing inflammation and promoting relaxation.

Here are some popular complementary therapies beneficial for menopause:

1. Acupuncture: Originating from traditional Chinese medicine, acupuncture involves

inserting thin needles into specific body points. Studies suggest its efficacy in reducing hot flashes and night sweats.

2. Massage Therapy: Relaxing massages are beneficial for stress management, muscle tension reduction, and overall well-being, with specific techniques tailored to alleviate menopausal symptoms.

3. Yoga: Combining physical postures, breathing exercises, and meditation, yoga is effective for stress management, enhancing sleep quality, and promoting relaxation, all of which benefit the menopause journey.

4. Tai Chi: This gentle exercise incorporates slow, graceful movements and deep breathing, improving balance, flexibility, and stress reduction, positively impacting menopausal experiences.

5. Meditation: Devoting a few minutes daily to focus on breath and quieting the mind effectively manages stress and induces relaxation, with various meditation techniques available for exploration.

## Key Considerations for Exploring Complementary Therapies

- ❖ Consult Your Doctor: Prior to initiating any new complementary therapy, seek advice from your physician to ensure safety and address potential medication interactions.
- ❖ Select Qualified Practitioners: Opt for experienced and licensed practitioners for any chosen complementary therapy.
- ❖ Exercise Patience: Consistency is key; allow time for complementary therapies to demonstrate their full benefits.
- ❖ Listen to Your Body: Monitor your body's response to each therapy, discontinuing if discomfort or adverse effects arise, and consulting your doctor promptly.

Incorporating complementary therapies into your menopause management fosters natural symptom alleviation, relaxation promotion, and overall well-being enhancement. The subsequent chapter will explore the potential benefits of integrating herbs and supplements into your menopause regimen.

## 9.2: Herbal and Supplemental Aids for Menopause

Nature offers a diverse array of remedies, and during menopause, many women turn to botanical resources for relief. However, it's imperative to approach herbal remedies with care and understanding. This section delves into commonly utilized herbs and supplements for menopause, outlining their potential advantages and risks. It's essential to underscore that this information does not replace professional medical advice, and consulting your physician before commencing any new herbs or supplements is paramount to ensure safety and avoid potential interactions with current medications.

**Grasping Herbal Solutions**

Herbs and supplements can complement your menopause management strategy, yet comprehending their mechanisms and expected outcomes is pivotal. Consider the following:

- **Not Instant Solutions:** Unlike pharmaceuticals, herbs and supplements may necessitate time before discernible effects manifest. Consistency and patience are crucial for evaluating efficacy.

- **Potential Side Effects:** While generally milder than pharmaceuticals, herbs and supplements may induce side effects. Thoroughly research potential side effects before initiating a new remedy, and discontinue use if adverse reactions occur.
- **Medication Interactions:** Certain herbs and supplements may interact with existing medications. Therefore, disclosing all contemplated supplements to your healthcare provider is imperative to mitigate potential complications.

**Exploring Common Herbal Remedies**

Let's delve into several prevalent herbs and supplements that might alleviate menopausal symptoms:

01. **Black Cohosh:**
Historically used for managing hot flashes and night sweats, black cohosh's efficacy varies among individuals. Caution is warranted, especially for those with liver issues or undergoing hormone replacement therapy.

02. **Evening Primrose**
Oil: Rich in fatty acids, evening primrose oil may alleviate vaginal dryness.

However, caution is advised due to potential interactions with blood thinners and certain seizure medications.

### 03. Red Clover:

Bearing estrogen-like compounds, red clover may alleviate symptoms like hot flashes and mood swings. However, its suitability for individuals with specific health conditions necessitates consultation with a healthcare provider.

### 04. Flaxseed:

Abundant in lignans with weak estrogenic properties, flaxseed may mitigate hot flashes and night sweats. Incorporating ground flaxseed into dietary staples offers a convenient approach.

### 05. Ashwagandha:

An adaptogenic herb with a history in Ayurvedic medicine, ashwagandha shows promise in managing stress and anxiety, prevalent concerns during menopause.

This list is not exhaustive, and various other herbs and supplements may address specific menopause symptoms. Conduct thorough research, engage in dialogue with your physician, and determine the best fit for your individual needs.

**A Cautionary Note: Prioritize Safety!**

While herbs and supplements offer natural alternatives for managing menopause symptoms, safety remains paramount. Additional considerations include:

- ❖ Source Quality: Procure herbs and supplements from reputable sources with stringent quality control measures.
- ❖ Adherence to Dosage: Abide by recommended dosages to avoid adverse effects, as surpassing these limits may yield unintended consequences.
- ❖ Exercise Patience: Allow sufficient time for herbs and supplements to exert their effects, recognizing that notable changes may require several weeks of consistent usage.

By approaching herbal remedies with prudence, knowledge, and under medical supervision, you can leverage nature's offerings to navigate the menopause journey with enhanced comfort and well-being.

# 9.3: Cultivating Mindfulness: Strategies for Stress Alleviation and Inner Harmony

The tumultuous emotional journey of menopause can present significant hurdles. In my personal experience, stress and anxiety often overwhelmed me, leading to restless nights and an overall sense of unease. However, embracing mindfulness became a potent tool in my arsenal for confronting these emotional challenges and discovering inner serenity during this transformative phase.

**Defining Mindfulness:**

Mindfulness entails attentiveness to the present moment devoid of judgment. It involves acknowledging thoughts, emotions, and bodily sensations in a non-reactive manner. By nurturing present-moment awareness, one can detach from negative thoughts and anxieties, fostering tranquility and inner equilibrium.

**The Advantages of Mindfulness Amid Menopause:**

Incorporating mindfulness practices into daily routines yields several benefits during menopause:

1. Stress Alleviation: Menopause often induces significant stress, and mindfulness serves as an effective coping mechanism. By concentrating on breath and present sensations, the body's relaxation response is activated, diminishing stress hormones and inducing a sense of calmness.
2. Enhanced Sleep Quality: Stress and anxiety frequently disrupt sleep patterns, a prevalent issue during menopause. Mindfulness practices prepare the mind and body for restful sleep by quieting mental chatter.
3. Emotional Regulation: Menopause's emotional rollercoaster can be challenging to navigate, but mindfulness enables observation of emotions without judgment, facilitating proactive responses over reactive negativity.
4. Augmented Self-Awareness: Mindfulness fosters self-awareness, aiding in identifying stress and anxiety triggers. Armed with this awareness, individuals can proactively implement strategies for managing triggers and preserving emotional well-being.

**Initiating Mindfulness Practices:**

Mindfulness is adaptable to all experience levels and can be seamlessly integrated into daily routines.

Consider these steps to embark on your mindfulness journey:

- Commence Gradually: Begin with brief mindfulness sessions daily, gradually increasing duration as comfort levels grow.
- Secure a Tranquil Space: Choose a serene environment free from distractions, such as a bedroom corner, a secluded outdoor spot, or an office during breaks.
- Center on Breathing: Direct focus inward by closing eyes or softening gaze, centering attention on the breath's rhythm. If distractions arise, gently guide focus back to the present without judgment.
- Embrace the Process: Mindfulness is a continual practice, not an endpoint. Accept fluctuations in focus without discouragement, gently steering attention back to the present moment.

Integrating mindfulness into my routine has been transformative. Even brief morning deep-breathing sessions instill centeredness and bolster stress management throughout the day. During heightened anxiety episodes, guided meditation apps offer solace, guiding me through calming visualizations to quell mental turbulence.

**Exploring Mindfulness Techniques:**

Explore various mindfulness techniques to identify those resonating with your needs:

- **Meditation:** Diverse meditation styles cater to individual preferences, from breath-focused meditation to loving-kindness meditation, offering avenues for self-exploration.
- **Mindful Movement:** Activities like yoga, tai chi, or mindful walking fuse physical movement with mindfulness, fostering relaxation and present-moment awareness.
- **Body Scan Meditation:** This technique involves systematically scanning the body for sensations without judgment, aiding in tension release.

Mindfulness is a journey marked by progress. Embrace patience and celebrate incremental advancements. By incorporating mindfulness into daily life, inner peace can be cultivated, stress managed effectively, and the emotional turbulence of menopause traversed with greater ease.

# CHAPTER 10: EMBRACING TRANSFORMATION AND HARNESSING INNER POWER

Menopause is often depicted as a period of decline – the conclusion of fertility and the fading of youth. Yet, what if we reimagined it? Picture menopause as an opportunity for profound transformation, a gateway to embarking on a potent new chapter enriched with wisdom, resilience, and renewed purpose. This chapter centers on honoring yourself – embracing metamorphosis and seizing control of your authority as you traverse this exhilarating phase of life.

## 10.1: Rethinking Menopause: A Phase of Growth, Not Diminishment

Menopause, an intrinsic biological phase experienced by all women, heralds certain physical alterations. However, resist allowing these changes to define your journey. Menopause signifies not the termination of your well-being, vigor, or femininity. Rather, it can signify liberation – a moment to discard societal pressures and embrace your genuine essence.

Throughout my personal journey of menopause, adjustments were inevitable. Yet, I've come to perceive it as a period of self-discovery. I no longer feel constrained by unattainable beauty standards; instead, I prioritize pursuits that ignite joy and fulfillment. Menopause, to me, catalyzed a profound surge in self-assurance and liberation.

**The Potential of Reframing**

The key to fostering a positive menopausal experience lies in the lens through which it is viewed. Here are strategies to reframe your outlook and commemorate the evolution accompanying this transition:

- ❖ Highlight Your Fortitudes: Menopause heralds a treasure trove of life acumen and sagacity. Acknowledge your strengths and achievements. You've weathered storms, forged connections, and evolved as an individual. Embrace this internal resilience and wisdom as you progress.

- ❖ Embrace Body Appreciation: Your body is a formidable and adaptable entity. It has shepherded you through life's odyssey and continues to do so. Foster body positivity and self-kindness. Seek ways to nurture and engage your body in activities that promote well-being.

❖ Cultivate a Mindset Shift: Instead of fixating on perceived losses, channel your focus towards the prospects that lie ahead. What sparks your enthusiasm? What novel adventures beckon? Foster a mindset of growth and welcome the avenues for personal advancement.

Reframing my outlook has been transformative. Rather than dreading transitions, I've begun to perceive them as natural progressions. I've accentuated my strengths, celebrated my body's resilience, and redirected my attention towards enticing new prospects. This shift in perspective has bestowed upon me a newfound tranquility and empowerment.

## 10.2: Formulating a Vision for the Future and Embracing Novel Opportunities

View menopause as a blank canvas – an invitation to craft a vision for the future that resonates with your current values and aspirations. Here are tactics to assist you in painting this dynamic tableau:

→ **Contemplate Your Passions:** What ignites your enthusiasm? Which endeavors bring you profound satisfaction? Dedicate time to introspection. Catalog your passions and interests – ranging from artistic pursuits to globetrotting adventures.

→ **Establish Objectives:** Once your passions are identified, transform them into tangible objectives. These objectives can encompass various scopes, whether personal or professional, grand or modest. Defined objectives furnish a sense of purpose and trajectory as you navigate this fresh phase.

→ **Embrace Novel Pursuits:** Embrace the unfamiliar without trepidation. This juncture is an opportune moment to probe uncharted territories and kindle your inquisitiveness. Contemplate embarking on a solitary voyage, acquiring a new skill, or committing to a cause close to your heart.

Crafting a vision board facilitated the visualization of my future aspirations. Adorned with depictions representing my passions – traversing the globe, engaging in a local writing enclave, and cherishing moments with cherished ones – this visual aid motivates me to persevere and seize the thrilling prospects on the horizon.

Remember, camaraderie abounds on this journey. Engage with fellow women traversing menopause. Support groups or virtual communities serve as invaluable wellsprings of knowledge, fellowship, and communal narratives.

## Embrace the Metamorphosis

Menopause heralds a metamorphic phase – an opportunity to embrace personal evolution and redefine the essence of feminine strength and vitality. By reimagining this transition, assuming responsibility for your well-being, and prioritizing your fervors, you can stride into the ensuing chapter of your life with assurance, resolve, and an empowered spirit of celebration.

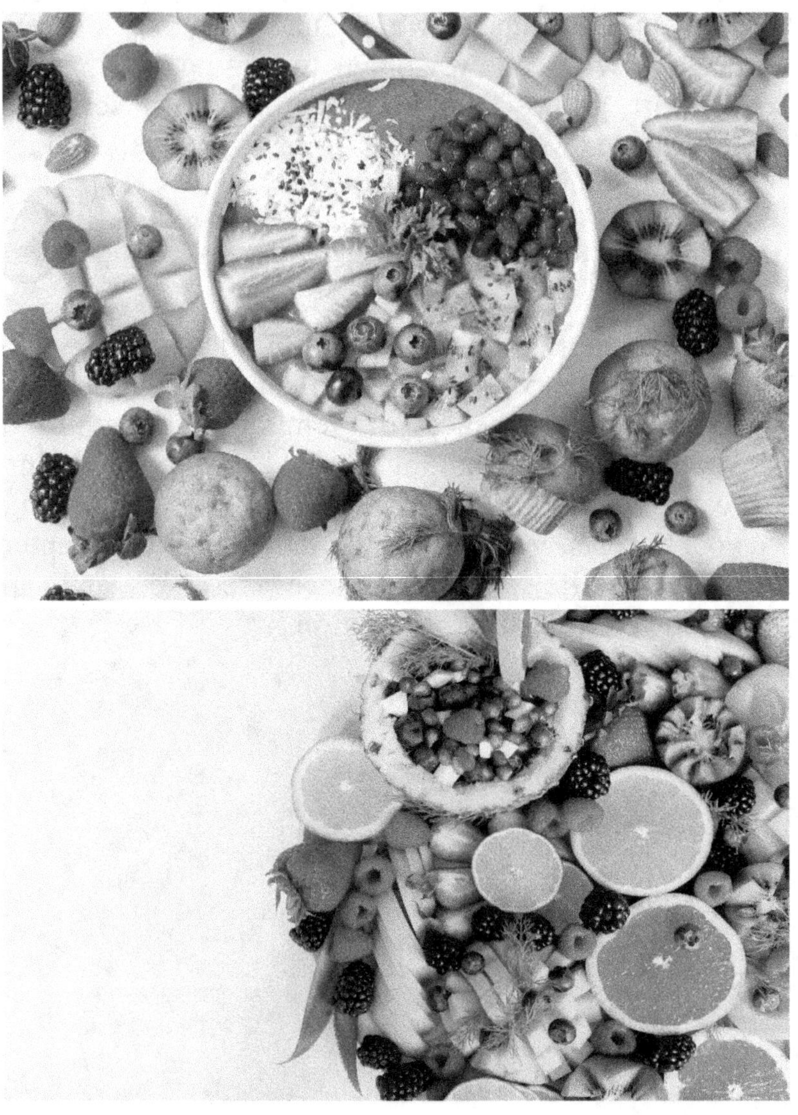

# CONCLUSION

You've reached the culmination of our journey together, exploring the intricate landscape of menopause and its profound impact on your physical, emotional, and social well-being. Throughout these chapters, we've delved into the scientific underpinnings of menopause, examined diverse approaches to symptom management, and heralded the transformative potential inherent in this transition.

As a fellow traveler on this path, I confidently affirm that menopause is not a phenomenon to dread but rather one to embrace wholeheartedly. It signifies a natural progression, an opportunity to step into a fresh chapter overflowing with promise.

This book has furnished you with the knowledge and resources essential for navigating the changes accompanying menopause. Yet, remember, your most potent asset is yourself. Your inner fortitude, adaptability, and sagacity serve as guiding beacons as you forge ahead.

A Concluding Note of Encouragement: Seize Your Power, Commemorate Your Voyage

Assert your power – the power of your voice, your decisions, and your distinctive viewpoint. Now is the time to prioritize self-nurturance, delve into your passions, and embrace the woman you've evolved into. Don't hesitate to realign your priorities, establish fresh objectives, and embark on exhilarating adventures.

Celebrate your journey! Menopause epitomizes the remarkable resilience and strength inherent in the female form. Recognize your triumphs, embrace the evolution of your body, and foster self-compassion throughout the process.

Reflecting on my own odyssey, I'm imbued with gratitude for this transformative passage. While menopause has presented its share of hurdles, it has also bestowed upon me an unforeseen sense of liberation and empowerment. I'm eager for the myriad possibilities that lie ahead, and I trust you share this sentiment.

## <u>Acknowledgments</u>

I extend heartfelt gratitude to you for selecting this book as your companion on your menopause expedition. My aspiration is that the information and perspectives imparted herein empower you to traverse this transition with assurance, insight, and a spirit of empowered jubilation. Remember, you are not traversing this path in solitude.

A vibrant community of women stands ready to support and uplift one another during menopause. Engage with these women, exchange experiences, and exalt each other's resilience and vigor.

May the subsequent chapter of your life brim with vitality, contentment, and a renewed sense of mission. Embrace the metamorphosis, celebrate yourself!

**Bonus Tip:** While this book has furnished a comprehensive overview of menopause, remember that each woman's journey is singular. Don't hesitate to solicit personalized guidance and support from your healthcare provider as you navigate this transition.

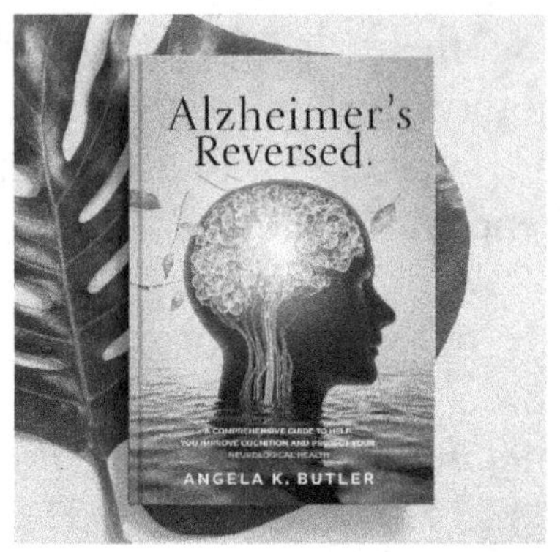

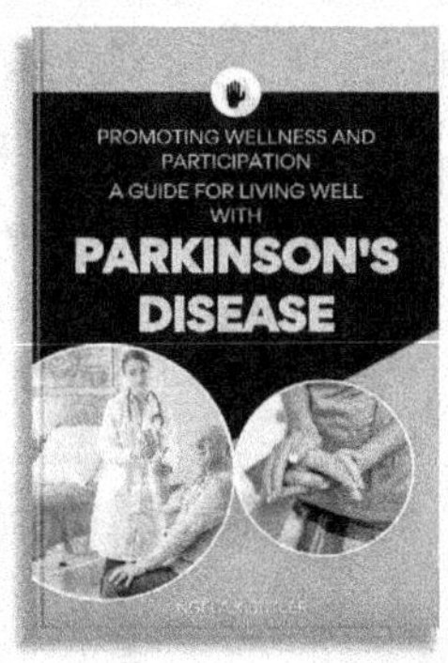

If you liked this book, be sure to check out my other books, **"ALZHEIMER'S REVERSED:** A COMPREHENSIVE GUIDE TO HELP YOU IMPROVE COGNITION AND PROTECT YOUR NEUROLOGICAL HEALTH"** and **"PROMOTING WELLNESS AND PARTICIPATION:** A GUIDE FOR LIVING WELL WITH PARKINSON'S DISEASE" available on Amazon.